FORENSIC MEDICINE IN INDIA

FORENSIC MEDICINE IN INDIA

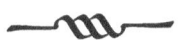

AN INTRODUCTION

ARNEET ARORA

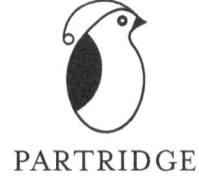

PARTRIDGE

To order additional copies of this book, contact
Partridge India
000 800 10062 62
orders.india@partridgepublishing.com

www.partridgepublishing.com/india

CONTENTS

Dedication vii

Acknowledgements... ix

Preface xi

Introduction...xv

Forensic Medicine in India: how it is
    and what it includes 1

My interest in Forensic Medicine 6

The undergraduate Forensic Medicine........................... 13

Post graduation in Forensic Medicine........................... 23

Court evidences 30

Special cases..45

Critical analysis of the subject and future directions...... 64

List of photographs and illustrations

Illustrations

1. A student with a book associating the work in Forensic Medicine.
2. Autopsy being performed in the Mortuary.
3. Stretcher with a body on it.
4. Travelling in the bus right next to a goat
5. Sketch of the District and Sessions Court Bhopal.

DEDICATION

The book is dedicated to Prof B P Dubey for being who he has been for all these years.

Acknowledgements

I would like to thank Mr Ashwin Pandya for the sketches in the book. He is an acknowledged artist and his skills are commendable. He can draw a sketch to a narration and make real, the abstract invisible image described to him. The sketches match the expectation of the person for whom he creates and customises. His spontaneity translates into a speed making the process almost as interesting to watch as a time lapse photograph.

My friends and colleagues have encouraged me to share my experiences and the book is primarily because they could convince me to have it published.

Preface

India as a country is unique in how it works and only people who have been here awhile can really decode its essence. Doing Autopsies or post mortem (as it is commonly referred here), which involves dissecting the dead body and looking into dead remains of a person, is a skill and a job unlike any other. Autopsy in India, is a distinct experience and I hope to show you in these few pages how it was 25 years ago and how it is evolving over time.

Investigation of suspicious deaths or crimes or the inquest is done by the police in India. Inquest by magistrate is done in a few specific cases, for example deaths in police custody, where exhumation is required, cases of dowry deaths, etc. Medicolegal autopsy is done as part of the inquest by the inquesting agency. Autopsy is done on receiving the requisition from the Police. Autopsy starts after the dead body is identified by the police. The report of the autopsy is given by the autopsy surgeon to the police. Police may forward samples for investigation to the forensic scientists. Autopsy surgeon can also forward samples for further investigation to the forensic laboratories or forensic scientists. Forensic science and autopsy go hand in hand and together determine the technological status of investigation. Each country develops its level of skill, rate of upgradation of services and administration of justice based on these findings.

Forensic Medicine as a subject is not a hot favourite with medical graduates for a variety of reasons. There are very few institutes which offer post graduation in Forensic Medicine and yet at times these positions remain vacant. The clinical subjects are favoured by medicine graduates. Forensic Medicine because it alienates from hospital and clinical work, requires the post graduate to conduct autopsies and visit the courts frequently for court evidence, intimidates the graduates. Most students will admit that they find the subject interesting and challenging, but not many opt for it for allied reasons. The job of a Forensic expert in India has its own challenges and responsibilities. It is an interesting world and lately with some young, driven and intellectually motivated having joined the specialty, it seems to be moving with new speed, addressing the sub specialities and integrating better with forensic scientists, people in law and other medical branches.

When I was about to enter the world of Forensic Medicine, I came across the book 'Autopsy' by Dr Bernard Knight based on the professional life and values of Dr Milton Helpern of USA and included details about the illustrious cases he was involved in. The book was so honest and clear about what a Forensic expert does and the frame of mind required for the same, that it helped to clarify quite diverse confusions regarding this field. But they were the details of a Medical Examiner's work in USA, decades earlier, and hence quite different. However, it is such a well written book that it takes the interest level of the reader a level higher.

Reading medical thrillers by Robin Cook and Arthur Hailey and the court thrillers by Erle Stanley Gardner with Perry Mason as the protagonist and a lawyer, helped me understand the intricacies mentioned in the book

'Autopsy'. In India, one opts directly for Forensic Medicine for post graduation, while in many countries it is a super specialisation, which a post graduate in Pathology opts for. In India, Forensic Medicine is taught to undergraduates and has hundred hours allotted to it. It requires an undergraduate to see autopsies and learn to make reports for medicolegal cases related to injuries, sexual assaults and age estimation. The undergraduates do not visit the court which does not complete their picture or concept on application of the medicolegal work. The undergraduates also are overwhelmed with other subjects and clinical training during this time and this perhaps does not permit them to experience and form a complete picture of the role of the subject.

The idea for writing this book is to provide preliminary information to people interested in Forensic Medicine, who want to know what and how a Forensic expert is trained and what the work of a Forensic expert involves here in India. I have been in Forensic Medicine since 1993 when I registered for post graduation course, then worked at a few places, attended various conferences, met some of the big names in the specialty, compared and saw mortuaries in other countries, given evidence in court in several cases, seen a wide variety of autopsy cases and had the privilege of discussing and having guidance from several accomplished people in Forensic Medicine. It seemed appropriate to me to share in short a few experiences and /or lessons from these experiences in the form of this book.

It is my first experience in writing a book of this sort and hence would have several shortcomings. I have gone ahead with the book anyway giving in to the desire of sharing what I have shared in this book.

Introduction

Dear readers,

The book is meant for people who want to know what practice of Forensic Medicine is like in India. It brings out essence of what one may expect to find if one is contemplating on being part of it. The technical details and technical analysis is deliberately avoided and refrained from. There is ample opportunity in the branch to make a difference to how the world works and to ensure justice to aggrieved or marginalised people. It also has potential for name and fame for the Forensic person, should a person imbibe and develop the skill and combine with art of presentation in court.

The book will describe the work of a Forensic pathologist involved in autopsies of legal significance in India and that clinical Forensic Medicine is also part of his work.

It will provide information regarding the subject to the people interested in knowing about Forensic Medicine and to those interested in pursuing a career in the subject. The information given is limited to what the subject is in India. I hope the language is simple and easy to understand.

Details of the autopsy findings, its interpretations and submissions in courts have been purposely avoided. These things are best learnt when working and being involved in the cases. Besides, this book is not supposed to be anything close to a textbook. What has been attempted to convey here is what this job involves, how exciting it can be and what 'highs' it can make you feel and reach.

The infrastructure and facilities for medicolegal autopsy varies across the country. The description of the mortuary and its related facilities refer to the mortuary at Bhopal, located in central part of India, which is relatively quite well developed in comparison to the services available in other parts of the country.

It is an honest and candid description and at no place covered by any false pretences or information, to the best of my knowledge.

The book is divided into 7 chapters: the first deals with how Forensic Medicine is practiced in India, the second has autobiographical content in relation to the subject, the third deals with the exposure of a medical undergraduate to the subject, fourth to the issues of training and learning of the subject by a postgraduate, fifth demystifies court evidences faced by Forensic people and its challenges, sixth with short incomplete descriptions of cases seen by the author and the seventh chapter on overall analysis of the subject in terms of its practical application and limitations in the current context. The chapters are independent of each other and can be read in any sequence the reader may be interested in.

I hope the contents of the book are understandable and interesting to you and at the end you feel that it was worth the read.

Forensic Medicine in India: how it is and what it includes

Forensic Medicine in India implies a combination of what in most countries is considered as three separate entities Forensic Pathology, Forensic Medicine and Toxicology.

Forensic Pathology deals exclusively with autopsies done for Medicolegal purposes, what is commonly referred to as 'post mortem' in all cases of accidents, suicides, homicides, sudden deaths and suspicious deaths.

Clinical Forensic Medicine implies living human beings which are examined for some medicolegal purpose like examination of injuries, with history of sexual assault as victim or accused or for estimation of age.

Toxicology is the study of poisons, their identification, types, causes, effects, treatment and implications. It can commonly be divided into three sub groups: clinical toxicology including the signs and symptoms of poisoning and their treatment, Forensic Toxicology including study of poisons with medicolegal significance for example homicidal, or suicidal poisoning or mass poisoning and third sub group being toxicology of substances used as drugs of abuse.

Forensic Medicine although was introduced to me in my second undergraduate year of Medicine in 1988, I started knowing it better as a post graduate student since 1993. People, at least in India, find it difficult to accept that cutting or rather dissecting dead bodies and discussing how and why the person died would be a profession one opts for. It becomes further difficult to accept when they realise that not too rarely one conducts the autopsy on decomposed bodies. But it is such a challenging mental exercise that to me it is perfectly understandable as a profession by choice. The why and how of death of the deceased is also not over in the Mortuary. It may involve visit to the site, the place where the body was found and lot of investigations. The facts and their interpretation are then sent to the court. The doctors are summoned to the court where they deposit their evidence and are cross examined on their reports and inferences.

The process of autopsy with context to the history of the case is engrossing very often. The analysis of autopsy findings after conducting the autopsy is a unique intellectual exercise. It is a scientific process whereby one postulates the various options and processes which could have caused the outcome observed. It is a rich mix of knowledge of Medicine, Psychology, Physics and Law which helps the Forensic person to arrive at an opinion and express with appropriate words. The choice of words to be used in the autopsy report and the meaning it would imply in the court is a knowledge gradually acquired with time and experience. The sense of fulfilment on an autopsy well done and the evidence well delivered in court is immense. The court is the place where science and art meet: the science of facts and probabilities with the art of presentation.

The assets of this branch are considered as drawbacks by a lot of people. Looking at the dead, dissecting and inspecting their organs and writing a report or opinion which would be discussed and debated in court and perhaps involve a gruelling cross examination by a lawyer is the work of a Forensic Pathologist. This is a mechanical expression of the work done by the Forensic pathologist. In reality, it is a challenging process, exciting at times. To witness the autopsy and to understand the process of death in an individual is a privilege. It is like a puzzle where pieces are picked, gathered and placed together and then a pattern begins to emerge. This exercise evolves the thinking process to log back into the past and visualise the action in the past by the effect seen in the present. The analysis will be subject to doubts, suspicion and disbelief. The results of investigations may add evidence and support to the chronology of events but the degree of certainty is difficult to ascertain. It is amidst this mix of evidence, the degree of specificity of the findings and the validity of the interpretation derived, that a cross examination in court of law can be a test of knowledge, wits, personality and communication skills. No science is perfect and no investigation exact. A test we consider infallible today may have its inaccuracies detected tomorrow. DNA fingerprinting, a modern technology used as a final word in several cases is being questioned for its subjectivity at times and is not beyond suspicion. With subjectivity and bias creeping inadvertently in addition to deliberate or manipulative interpretation, audit of all reports and investigations within a reasonable time from unrelated distant agency is perhaps the only solution.

The application of Forensic Pathology in criminal cases, facilitating differentiation of manner of death, providing clarity on cause of death in hospital deaths and providing clues in investigation of suspected poisoning cases seem more than enough reasons to promote the subject and its use, but ironically it was never promoted as it deserved. Forensic Pathology is the domain of the government and no private institution or college can promote its cause.

There is no apex institute in the country involved and dedicated to Forensic Pathology and all its allied specialties as the referral institute for Forensic cases. The allied specialties include Forensic Medicine, Toxicology, Forensic Radiology, Forensic Odontology, Forensic Anthropology and Forensic Sciences including DNA fingerprinting. The culture of work, training facilities and integration of sub specialties in Forensic Pathology and allied subjects needs to be developed and evaluated in the country.

The work of a Forensic Pathologist is sometimes seen with awe and admiration for it is an unusual job and its true spirit still unravelled.

The first time that someone watches an autopsy being done is an experience no one forgets. Since the age of 6-7 years, the curiosity about what is inside us and how does it look, exists. Children are full of ideas and thoughts they have gathered from people around them. I have a couple of times demonstrated to children 10 to 12 years old, the inside of the human body at autopsy demonstration. When the children themselves are interested in looking at the inside of the human body, they do not get scared, rather they expressed that they wanted to feel the lungs and the heart. They were also happy to see the varied colour of organs, the bright yellow of fat, the reddish brown of liver and the stomach as a bag. If we could only convey to our children, in the true spirit of things, how beautifully designed our inner bodies are, show them its picture, explain its working, perhaps let them touch, if possible, the various organs, they would not only feel proud of their beautiful gift called body, but would also never smirk at body parts and rather spontaneously respect human tissues and would like to understand its working, in greater depth. There are children who believe that brain is in liquid or colloid form and they are surprised to see it as a solid organ, white to grey in colour. Some of the children also believed that the inside of our bodies is not clean and when they do look inside, they are pleasantly surprised to see various organs.

My interest in Forensic Medicine

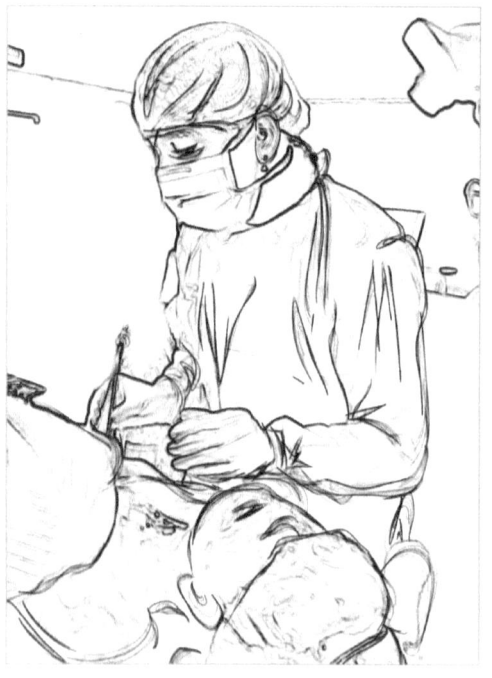

The place I did my graduation in late 1980s was Gandhi Medical College, a government medical college which also had a Medico Legal Institute as part of Home department, attached to it. The Medical colleges usually are referral centres for medico legal autopsies, conducting autopsies on dead bodies from around the area. Medico legal Institute was the referral centre for the entire state. Forensic persons in both the Medical college and the Medico legal Institute were housed on the same floor of the college building, sharing a common reception, common Mortuary, common autopsy record and a common duty roster. In short, functionally the two diverse working units worked as one. That had advantages for both beyond the predictable administrative and financial advantages. Forensic persons in Medical college were involved with undergraduate and postgraduate teaching. Forensic persons in Medico legal Institute would get expert opinion cases referred to them from all over the State of Madhya Pradesh. The Medico legal Institute had Forensic Dentistry, Forensic Anthropology, Forensic Photography, Forensic Histopathology, Forensic Entomology, Forensic Toxicology units and a Diatom Lab. This institute had started way back in 1977 and was visualised and planned by Dr Heeresh Chandra, who became its Founder Director. He did not compromise on infrastructure and human resource in any way and ensured that people with required qualification were selected for various technical posts. With time their exposure to different cases provided them with a rich experience and they became an authority in their area of work. At the time that it started the best of equipments available were procured to have reliable results of best quality possible. Facilities for gas chromatography, liquid chromatography, high end microscope with fluorescent microscopy, Anthropology instruments, autopsy instruments with electric saw, etc were all available.

There were about 10 Forensic Pathologists available in late 80s jointly between the Medicolegal Institute and

Gandhi Medical College. The annual autopsy rate had reached between 2,500 to 3,000 autopsies and then there were clinical Forensic Medicine cases of age estimation, injuries and sexual assault. There was enough work to keep everyone busy.

As an undergraduate student, I was in awe of the Museum which had a series of foetus of different ages in bottles, specimens of external and internal injuries, snakes, poisons, skull and other bones, weapons, X rays plates showing injuries and process of ossification, photographs and charts. At the entrance to the museum, a hanging mannequin greeted me and an articulated complete human skeleton right in its centre stared at me. It was scary the first time but quite admirable subsequently for one could appreciate the detailing on the hanging mannequin in terms of its head being tilted opposite to the knot, saliva coming out from the angle of mouth opposite to the knot and feet stretched and straightened.

We were demonstrated about 10 autopsies during under graduation period and for each autopsy demonstration, four of us were asked to wear gloves and participate in the dissection. It was for the first time that we were seeing a real case with a history provided by the police and the opinion after the autopsy being looked up to for further information. It was exciting to see how the opinion by the autopsy surgeon was intently listened by the police officer and decide onward direction of investigation. The practicals included those on Forensic Entomology, examination of clothings and weapon, Forensic Osteology and Histology. In Forensic Entomology demonstration class, I was literally dumbstruck by how much information an expert on insects working in Forensic field could gather from insects found on dead body. He could suggest whether the dead body has been moved after death and give a reasonable range for time of death in decomposed bodies where the body was seen days or weeks after death. The toughest I found then was forensic anthropology, which is primarily examination of bones and giving an opinion after examination. The exhaustive number of bones does not make it any easier! Forensic samples of bones in real life are complex. There may be an incomplete set of bones or bones of more than one person mixed. To make it more complex, there may be intact bones or pieces of bones. There may be findings on bones that are significant and then those have to be documented and opinion drawn based on the findings.

I liked the subject as an undergraduate and contemplated a career in it. The reactions and disapproval from family and friends to this were much stronger than I had anticipated. I decided to explore the subject deeper and practically to be sure that I would be comfortable with it. I created an opportunity for myself during the third year of the MBBS (Medicine graduation) course itself. It was of course not a suggested or approved way!

A rural camp organised by Community and Family Medicine (then called Preventive and Social Medicine) for two weeks was compulsory for all undergraduates. I was also beginning to realise around that time that the desire to learn clinical skills and the clinical approach did not appeal my intellect. It was a challenge I did not want to be part of. I also felt the limitation of clinical subjects in demonstrating certainty of diagnosis. This of course was not true as I can see it now. It was my bias and lack of clinical skills which made me believe it at that time.

In contrast, autopsy offered more clarity by direct examination of organs and their abnormality, that is, macro pathology (pathology visible by naked eye without the aid of a microscope). The freedom to explore all organs in any way that one prefers seemed to permit intellectual freedom and analysis and felt like a tempting offer. h. Inspite of one's skills and experience, even with all possible efforts there are times when no pathology or cause of death is apparent at autopsy. It may feel like a dead end to the explorations done. But this is the real story which lot of pathologists face and it is discomforting and unrealistic sometimes to the court and even to the police. But then that is another story.

To continue with my story of undergraduate years, I did not go to the rural camp and instead decided to explore the possibility of observing day to day work of Forensic department. Those were the days that short term observer ship, short term fellowship, etc were not known at least to most of us as students. There were no formal documents for it and no permissions. When I think back now and recall over the years, I realise that no one as an undergraduate usually opted to work in Forensic Medicine and I was almost immediately accepted and taken in. I was not looking for any certificate of experience or training and was thrilled with the spontaneous permission granted. For the two weeks, including Sunday, I would reach the Forensic department at 10 am, start with attending an autopsy or two or a Medicolegal case or bone examination and then watch the reports or opinions drawn based on the observation. I would volunteer to write the rough notes, sketches showing burns and injuries, help in writing short reports for the autopsy which included the opinion. The Faculty found it convenient to dictate to me while I wrote. Those were the days when computers were non existent and everything was written on the forms which were kept available. I also volunteered to be the female witness when examination of female for age estimation, injury examination with or without sexual assault was being done. Everyone in the department was quite supportive and open to interaction and discussion. To me these experts seemed to handle complex cases with ease and control knowing exactly what to look for, how to mention it and predict questions and controversies which could arise in court later. What was particularly impressive, was how everyone was willing to show me what they were doing, explaining how they conduct an examination and include me in all the discussions and debates of the case. I was also allowed to go to the court with them, a couple of times. Most of the Faculty (including Senior Faculty) had scooters (two wheelers), unlike today when most junior doctors too have a car. Those were a little different times in many ways and the Faculty giving rides to students on scooter was unheard of. When I think back, I feel absolutely thankful that they seemed to be above all such norms and were so open to teaching and imparting all that they thought I might begin to understand. It takes a few times of visiting the court and hopefully with different people to understand how the courts work and how the attitude and response of expert witness account given by a doctor makes a difference to the case. They were able to convey and make me understand the importance of maintaining confidentiality and how careful one has to be in discussing information considered as sensitive, as it can create misunderstanding and unnecessary issues. This whole experience opened my mind to the practical aspects of the subject and affirmed to me that I liked all that the subject included.

I think it is a good idea to work and see before hand where you want to work eventually to rule out any rude shock one may otherwise walk into. Here again, the time of two weeks or more (if possible) would be appropriate. This trend in other countries is followed even by school going children, where they explore two or more options over vacations in last 3 to 4 years of their school. The school going children have enough time to explore and find their calling when exposed to several options. As undergraduates if we explore a few branches of Medicine, our own choices become clear to us. Some of us can find our passion, making life so much simpler.

The school days and to a limited extent, the college days that I did my bit of reading fiction and nonfiction in Hindi and in English, the books I read were the books that were available. Enid Blyton books dominated children's literature then and she was the first author we would invariably fall in love with. For some reason, I am still not sure how or why, I had at home almost the entire collection of Erle Stanley Gardner's series with Perry Mason the criminal lawyer as the protagonist. Agatha Christie books with Hercule Poirot and Miss Maple, Arthur Hailey, Robin Cook and Sherlock Holmes were the thriller books I read. I think they did play their role in arousing interest in investigation and how court testimony affects the outcome of the case, the role of evidence and admissible evidence, etc.

Somewhere along the way I began to think that this was my calling and nothing else would do.

The undergraduate Forensic Medicine

Graduation degree in Medicine is MBBS in India. There is a very competitive entrance examination to secure admission in a medical college for MBBS or to become a doctor. It is also one of the lengthiest, most demanding graduation course. The standard of education, infrastructure requirement and the qualification of faculty in medical colleges all over the country is determined by a Council called the Medical Council of India (MCI). Only a few elite colleges are beyond the purview of the Council.

In the first year of MBBS course, the new entrant is introduced to three subjects: Human Anatomy, Human Physiology and Biochemistry. Anatomy deals with study of various structures, organs and muscles of the body. To teach human anatomy dissection of dead human bodies is required. For this, the donated dead bodies are kept immersed in formalin tanks. These are brought out each day from the tank and dissected by a small group of about 6 to 8 students. The area they explore on dissection is the one taught to them in theory lecture the same day. It amounts to almost verifying what is taught and consolidating in memory the relative position of various structures in the body. They are thus introduced to dead body, but this dead body is remarkably different from what is seen later in Forensic Medicine autopsy demonstration.

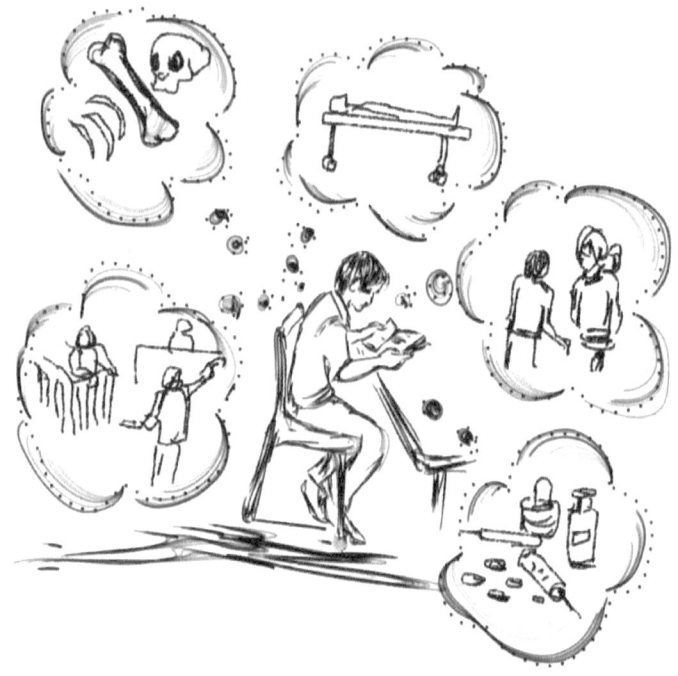

In the second year of under graduation, the subject Forensic Medicine and Toxicology is introduced and continues for about one and half years along with other para clinical subjects. The students devote about four hours per day to clinical subjects and about the same time to para clinical subjects. In Forensic Medicine, the students are taught about legal and ethical aspects of medical practice, the legal importance of examination in the so-called Medicolegal cases and how the knowledge of Medicine is applied for legal purposes.

It is one of the most crucial time, when all theoretical knowledge is beginning to see where it is likely to be applied and how. It is now a step up to their practical life, where they begin to visit wards and out patient departments, start integrating knowledge of Anatomy, Physiology and Biochemistry with laboratory reports and understanding principles of prescription of drugs to patients. The student has to correlate and integrate these subjects and form an integrated concept of various forms of ill health, how it presents and what should be its treatment. This is quite a challenge.

Amidst this demanding course, Forensic Medicine is a special subject which is connected to all the subjects yet different from them all. It forms a bridge, a liaison between two major professions, medicine and law. It is as diverse and interesting as life itself, yet deals with the dead too; a subject teaching and demonstrating how to apply grey areas of medicine to law. Law at first, seems to demand evidence and explanation in black and white, working with the grey(s) of life and health, addressing also issues of death and crime.

Forensic Medicine has a relatively objective approach in looking at the autopsy findings. It conveys these findings in the report and in the courts in a manner appropriate to meet the legal demands of the case in a language understandable to persons not acquainted with the medical terminology. Persons trained and working in Forensic medicine develop this acumen of extracting and presenting in court in a relevant way, the significance of clinical findings from perspective of the applicable law. It is an empowering skill gained steadily with increasing practical exposure.

A student usually looks at the subject from what they have known about it through the media, movies and thriller suspense or mystery books. Often it is exaggerated and incorrect representation of what can be reasonably achieved and how. Movies, television serials and fiction books have to incorporate dramatic elements sometimes not necessarily true for getting sufficient attention and readers. Reality is often different from the expectations then. For an undergraduate it is important to understand the limitations and requirements of his work when he graduates.

A graduate who starts working in government sector, at various primary and community health centres is expected to conduct autopsies independently, whatever may be his area of specialisation, if he is specialised. This also means that he or she has lot of court evidences to appear for and give information regarding their reports and opinion to the court in an appropriate way.

Understanding that this is the expectation, the education and learning must centre around it. A lot of practical real life autopsies or case work must be demonstrated along with court visits, wherever possible.

As a Medicine undergraduate, a student spends about 100 hours learning Forensic Medicine. Of these about 70 to 75 hours are assigned for theory lectures and about 25 to 30 hours for Practical demonstration. The theory lectures include the rules for autopsy, changes in body after death and their interpretation, the expected findings in autopsy in cases of trauma, poisoning, burns, hanging, strangulation, drowning, etc. What is equally important to know are signs of sexual assault and how to preserve evidence in such a case. Looking for signs of identification in case of unidentified bodies and preserving samples in cases of suspected poisoning are part of basic learning processes. The information on few poisons, Medicolegal importance of age, court procedure and medical negligence are also covered in theory lectures. Practical demonstration include autopsy demonstration, examination of weapons responsible for producing injuries, examination of hair to differentiate trauma by sharp or blunt weapon, examination of vaginal and seminal smear in cases of sexual assault and understanding the importance of insects in determining time since death in decomposed bodies. It also includes examination of clothing, bones and teeth, bone marrow for diatoms, plant poisons and examination of foetus for age estimation.

When the students are being introduced to the subject, they notice that practical examples to each thing they are taught and explained abound. There is however, one aspect to the subject which holds enigma and maximum curiosity, for which some cannot wait to experience and some feel an unwarranted dread for. It is the autopsy, where they would face a dead body with some medio-legal aspect which would require the person conducting the autopsy to either alleviate or substantiate facts related to the cause and manner of death. It would take varied time for each one of them to realize the quantum of skill and attitude which is needed to communicate with a dead body and gather information from it. It is an uphill task, like most other skilled works are. Initially, it is easier to get discouraged to follow it as it does not look like a lucrative or an attractive options. It is only when one has somewhat acquired the skill and has begun to exercise it, does one realize the 'kick' one gets of having solved a puzzle, of having inferred some significant finding in a case of homicide or providing some emotional solace to survivors and family members of a suicide victim by refuting some disturbing causes. It is hard to describe this fulfillment but it is there all the time.

A graduate is expected to conduct autopsies independently and hence as undergraduates they must learn the basics of conducting autopsy. They have to then write an opinion, preserving and sealing any samples of importance as required in a particular case. The Mortuary building and autopsy services vary widely all over the country. Medical Council of India (MCI), the organisation responsible for maintaining standard of medical education (amongst various other regulatory roles) prescribes the size of Mortuary, Faculty strength (number) and the minimum services or facilities available in each department. Inspections by MCI at regular intervals of all medical colleges in the country ensures that these standards are maintained. Whenever the services are found deficient, the permission of college to run the MBBS course (graduation course) becomes questionable, recognition of the college cancelled and further admission of students to MBBS course deferred. All colleges, government and private, now have the basic requirements fulfilled although the exposure to the autopsies and other practical aspects of the subject can and does vary markedly.

The first day when students watch their first autopsy, one or two might will feel nausea or giddiness or faintness. The first autopsy demonstration could mean one or two students dropping, fainting and leaving the mortuary with a handkerchief over their nose and mouth and making puking noises. Most of the students however watch it all with rapt attention and when they leave after seeing an autopsy, they have had a look they will remember. These are relatively fresh dead bodies as compared to the one they have seen for Anatomy dissection earlier. The dead body for anatomical dissection was embalmed and so nothing would flow, ooze or liquefy. Everything was relatively firm and fixed. The dead human body for autopsy was live a few hours ago usually and so the stomach contents may flow, fluids from brain and eyes flow, blood flows, pus flows and there may be liquefied organs.

Before starting the autopsy, the circumstances in which the body was found and history related to the case is told. The autopsy process is then demonstrated stepwise, the analysis and importance of the findings is assimilated and then interpretation and opinion writing discussed. When the process is repeated a few times with a variety of cases, they begin to understand the value of the autopsy findings and the science and art of opinion writing. Watching an autopsy is a unique experience and conducting it independently the first few times difficult. The balance of looking at it, with a purpose, to arrive at an opinion is what comes with time. Looking at the dead and analyzing the last moment of that life does make a person think and mature in a different way. Seeing the dead, emphasizes the contrast in life and enhances respect for human life.

In India, It is a rule to do complete autopsy, which means that all thoracic and abdominal organs and the brain would be examined in each case, whatever may be the cause of death. It is useful in many circumstances to assess the case completely. As for example, in case of death of a pedestrian in a road-traffic accident who dies of head injury, it may be interesting and informative to find that the deceased had cataract (lens of the eye which is normally transparent becomes opaque with age causing impaired vision) or that his coronaries (blood vessels of the heart) are almost completely occluded or blocked, which indicate the possible predisposing factors for the accident. As opposed to a complete autopsy, a partial autopsy is permissible legally in a few countries, where complete body is not examined rather, if a person is suspected of having died a death due to a coronary occlusion, the thoracic or chest cavity is opened, heart seen, removed from the body and its coronaries examined. If they are found to be occluded or blocked significantly, it is reported to be the underlying pathology responsible for the death of the person. But if no such pathology is found, it is reported as not being to coronary occlusion. Examination of other organs and finding the cause of death is not done in these circumstances

There are other legal requirements that the students must know about. It is included in what is called Medical Jurisprudence. This is technically legal aspect of medical practice. This includes all the legal principles that a doctor must know and follow in his practice after graduation. As for example he must know that he can take consent for examination from a patient when he is 12 years old or more. Before the patient is of 12 years, the consent for examination is taken from parents. If he does not know this rule and examines a 15 year old with consent from parents, his examination legally amounts to examination without consent. He can be charged for conducting the examination without consent. If he does not take written consent from a person before Medicolegal examination of that person, the consent is not valid.

A graduate must know his legal duty related to giving a death certificate. He must know when he is bound to issue a death certificate, when he cannot legally issue a death certificate and when he must ask the autopsy to be conducted. A graduate must know that it is his or her duty to preserve the stomach contents removed by gastric lavage (removing stomach contents through a tube pushed through mouth or nose) in a case of suspected poisoning.

This fluid must be handed over to the investigating agency. Failure to hand over the lavage sample may invite legal action against the doctor. Hence, they must also obtain receipt of handing over of the sample. They are also taught about who has to undergo a Medicolegal autopsy absolutely necessarily. For example, a newly married woman who has sustained extensive burns would have to be autopsied in the event of her death, whether she is hospitalised or non hospitalised after sustaining burns. Such deaths are called Dowry deaths and hold special significance in social and legal terms.

A graduate must also know how to receive the summon and attend the court. He or she must know what to preserve, the preservative to be used and receipt for handing over the preserved article to be received. There are so many legal principles and procedures a medical practitioner is expected to know and follow that Forensic Medicine has its hands full with what they want the undergraduate to necessarily become aware of. Ignorance of a rule is not accepted as defence by the court so that there is no alternative for a doctor to practice but with the knowledge of laws as applicable to him.

There are tricky situations in a doctor's career when he can be charged for negligence by the patient for reasons not directly related to him. This includes the actions done by people under him whom he is supposed to supervise at the time. An undergraduate is made aware about it under the term, vicarious responsibility. A doctor also must know that he cannot be held negligent if the patient has not taken his advice and the patient's action is pay responsible for the negative outcome. A doctor can easily negate it as a case of contributory negligence by the patient.

A doctor must know when the confidentiality of condition of the patient is to be maintained and when it has to be disclosed, which are known as principles of professional secrecy and privileged communication. Principles of Medical jurisprudence are essential for the medical practitioner to know and these are all part of subject of Forensic Medicine.

Post graduation in Forensic Medicine

A graduate in Medicine becomes eligible for the post graduation course in Forensic Medicine. There are fiercely competitive exams one has to score well in to be selected for a post graduation course. The selection relies entirely on the score in this objective examination. People who score well to be near the top can choose a subject, the others pick from the vacancy in different subjects available to them. In these circumstances, the inclination, attitude and talent of a student often lose their meaning. In an attempt to make the selection of students objective, to remove subjectivity and bias in selection, we have a system which disregards completely the interest and previous activities of the student which could have served as complementary criteria in selection of students in a particular specialty.

In many countries, one has to do a post graduation or a course in Pathology and then move on to Forensic Pathology. The subject Forensic Pathology in such circumstances acquires the status of a super specialty. This provides a firm background in Pathology including histopathology, which is the backbone of Forensic Pathology.

In India, the situation is quite different. Soon after graduation, one joins a three year post graduation course in Forensic Medicine. This broadly includes Forensic

Pathology, Clinical Forensic Medicine and Toxicology. In addition to these three, one must also get to know significant amount of Forensic Anthropology and Forensic Dentistry. In most medical colleges, not only the autopsy load in terms of number of autopsies is immense, but also the Clinical Forensic Medicine related cases of age estimation, injuries and sexual offences are brought in large numbers.

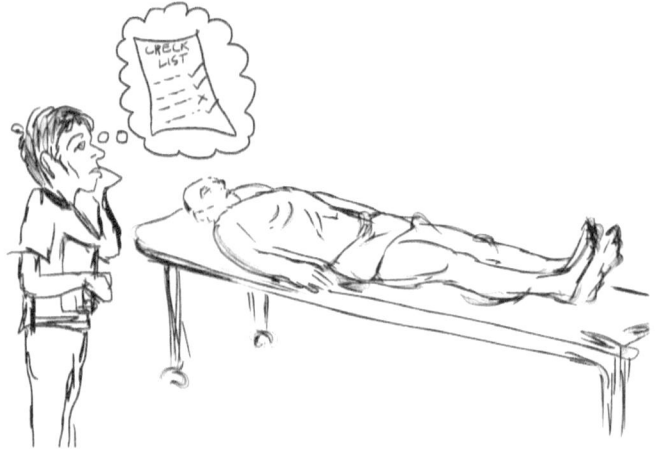

   The people in this subject have to interact with law and police departments during the course of their work. The communication with persons in these departments has to be correct, precise and easily understandable. The information and documents received by the police must be read well and understood before the examination of a Medicolegal clinical case or an autopsy begins. After the examination of the case and after an autopsy, the report is handed over to the police officer. This report is accompanied by samples of body tissues or fluids for further analysis, other articles like clothing, rope used as ligature, bullet or fingerprints for specific tests or reasons which must be explained to the investigating officer. In the court, the reports and the opinion have to be submitted and any findings which explain important conclusions must be explained well in the court. This is something one begins to observe and learn during his or her post graduation.

One of the basic and foremost expectation from a postgraduate is that he or she would be able to conduct autopsies independently and write the autopsy reports. He should also be able to answer questions appropriately when called as an expert in court evidences related to his cases. For this is required that he attends lot of autopsies and court evidences with faculty and senior students. It is then easy to understand the requirement of the court and the importance of cross examination. A centre which gets a large number of autopsies would thus have all types of cases and variety of court evidence related to these.

There is another important skill one gets introduced to and improves during post graduation. It is the teaching skill. As a postgraduate student, one is assigned practical demonstration classes for the under graduates. It is the opportunity to understand and try the basic tools of teaching. Answering the thoughts and questions raised by the undergraduates can sometimes stimulate one to think from a new perspective. Sometimes this is the only time one gets to catch up with skills for taking lectures one might have to, soon after post graduation.

This is also the first time one has to conduct research and present it as a thesis or dissertation. Although now few undergraduate students do small research projects, it is now as a postgraduate student that it becomes mandatory. Only when the research has been completed, written, published as a thesis and approved by two experts in the field is the student considered eligible for post graduation degree.

Forensic Medicine does not have enough well defined textbooks for post graduation level which has its major advantage and disadvantage. The advantage is that one explores the subject in several ways which enriches more than reading at one place from an author's perspective. The major disadvantage is that one has to invest a lot of time in this exploration. Thankfully, internet has revolutionised learning from what it was 20 to 25 years ago.

It is recommended for a person to understand and have an insight into the job requirements and have at least a rough idea of what this branch is all about. There was once a person who joined as postgraduate student in Forensic Medicine and on the first day attended the autopsy of a nine year old female who was strangulated after being raped. Taking the history of the case, looking at autopsy findings, and writing an opinion after discussion amongst the experts in the autopsy team, disturbed him so much that he dropped out from the course and never returned again. On a usual day there are autopsies, court evidences for some, autopsy follow up and documentation to be done by others so that it is sometimes not possible to brief about a case to a new student. Not clearly specifying our role or emphasising on what our focus is can disturb a yet to be accustomed person. One sometimes has to almost immediately get down to a case when it comes and not have time for psychological priming of the other. If the outlook can be formed before hand and one can see beyond the obvious trauma and focus on how the autopsy can provide evidence for commission of the crime, one can retain focus on the purpose and not lose balance.

A postgraduate student requires a good Forensic Pathology unit where a certain substantial number of autopsies of a variety of cases and an experienced trained faculty exist. In addition, if one were to look for a place which has a good unit in Toxicology and Clinical Forensic Medicine, there would be a very few organisations to choose from.

The service component and the academic component usually compete at an Institute and one of them is usually the priority at any given place. It just means that at some places the number of autopsies is big as compared to people doing the autopsy that getting the autopsies done, reports despatched and court evidences occupy the people predominantly. At other places where either the autopsies are not too many or people in enough number to handle the work, the people can focus on research, provided funding for research is available.

Attending conferences, seminars and workshops and presenting papers in conferences is expected from a post graduate. This becomes addictive for being a lively stimulant for updating one's information and knowledge levels in the future professional life too.

The centre in Bhopal where I enrolled for post graduation in 1993 had a caseload of about 2,200 to 2,500 cases per year including lot of referred cases from surrounding areas, decomposed bodies and practically all variety of Autopsy cases. With 7 persons at that time entrusted with autopsy work, each would get an average of about 300 to 350 autopsy cases per year. Then there would be Clinical Forensic medicine cases of age estimation, sexual assault and injury cases. The court evidences for these cases and autopsies would easily add up to about 8 to 10 cases in the local court and about 4 to 5 outside the district in each month for each person.

In the post graduation period in addition to learning the basic skills to conduct autopsy, write the autopsy reports, estimation of age, conducting a research towards thesis work, teaching the undergraduates, there are quite a few other things one must learn too. One very useful skill is taking photographs scientifically and appropriately, identified with autopsy number and date. For anything one needs to confirm later or for purpose of demonstration in court, the photographs can be very useful.

Handling documents of legal importance and storing them sometimes for decades makes one realise the importance of proper documentation. Medical colleges also handle referred autopsy cases from primary and community health centres. Police officers also get skeletonised human remains for examination. Knowledge of Forensic Anthropology and Dentistry is thus also required sometimes. The importance of collecting evidence and if possible its examination and report on it should be given by the Autopsy surgeon. When scalp hair or hair from elsewhere requires to be seen for differentiating sharp cut from crush injuries, collecting it, mounting it on the slide, examining, correlating and giving opinion is an exercise one learns only when one undertakes. This process in autopsy cases is similar to examination of vaginal smear in suspected sexual offence cases or examination of diatoms in suspected cases of drowning. Follow up of suspected poisoning cases helps to understand the importance of communication and correlation between autopsy person and the toxicologist without which chemical analysis of viscera may not yield significant results.

In cases of sudden deaths or when a pathology is suspected, histopathology examination must be undertaken and examination of slides must be done. In decomposed bodies when it is difficult to estimate the duration of death and entomological examination is often rewarding. All these require time and effort, but clarify the direction of investigation to be taken in future cases.

The clinical medicine ward sometimes send requests to Forensic medicine departments for opinion on Medicolegal cases. As a postgraduate, visit to the wards along with Forensic faculty helps to understand the dilemma a clinician faces in these cases.

Writing a report on expert opinion cases is an art with a protocol. Logical and well written expert opinion can help to solve the dilemma of courts or explain why the dilemma cannot be resolved.

One of the most important lesson a post graduate learns is that sometimes not having a clear opinion is an opinion. In these situations trying to give an opinion or trying to push an opinion may not be the best policy. Over opinionating however impressive or learned it may look, is unethical. One must draw conclusion only to the extent possible, logically and scientifically. That is practically one of the most difficult lessons to learn but one of the most essential too.

COURT EVIDENCES

Bhopal district court that I saw in the 1980s and 1990s was in Shahjahanabad area of Bhopal, housed in an old building with narrow corridors and the capacity of the building quite limited. It looked shabby and very badly maintained. It did not have enough parking area and the road to the court was quite narrow too. This would often lead to being in a traffic jam when going to the court. With two wheelers it was still manageable, but taking a car to the court was too uncomfortable and finding a place for parking, a bigger challenge.

The Bhopal district and session court moved into a new building and started its functioning there on 30th Oct 2004. It was located in new Bhopal area in an area where independent offices had recently emerged. It was the largest district court in Asia then built on 13 acres of land with cost of 10 crores. I am not sure whether it still is the largest district court of Asia or not. The building was truly grand. It felt like a court through and through and not a crouched up space, feeling ancient. It exudes vibrance and enthusiasm and somehow everything felt brisk, efficient and organized. Rules prohibiting photography of the building were not in force then and so when I visited the court a couple of days later, I could manage to take some photographs. The prohibition on photography was to follow a week later.

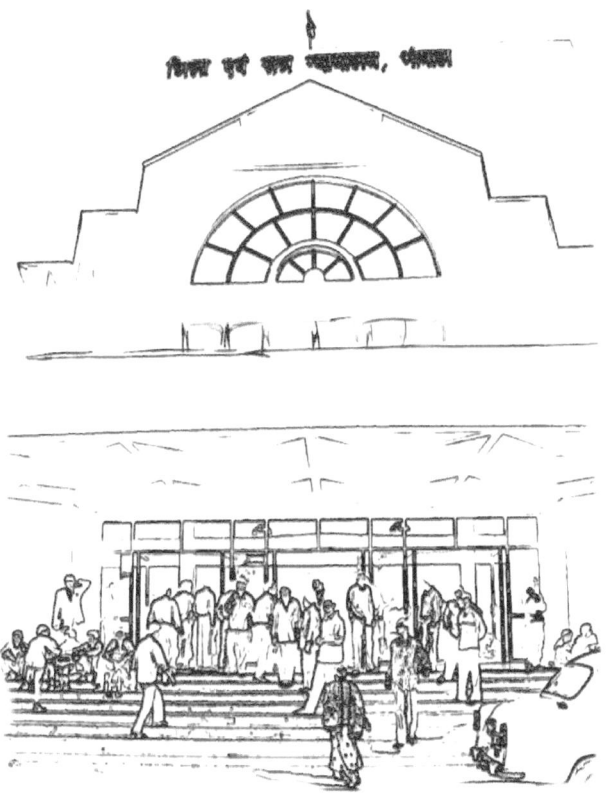

Court is finally the place where all that is observed, recorded and interpreted is brought to the fore-front. If it is conveyed logically with evidence to prove, it is accepted and otherwise rejected. It is the destination of all the relevant documents, witnesses – simple and expert, their deliberations and arguments, proofs and evidences.

The autopsy surgeon after a medicolegal autopsy, writes down the six page autopsy report which includes all the findings seen in the body externally and internally. This report form is the standard form in Madhya Pradesh state and varies from state to state in India. The writing of the report is an art and science both – it should technically explain all the relevant findings, be complete and clear and yet be understandable for the purpose of court. Some of our reports are accompanied with sketches showing mechanical or physical injuries, thermal injuries, pattern of injuries or frequency and extent of coronary occlusion. The sketch is just the outline of human body in 2D showing the front and the back. In cases of multiple physical or mechanical injuries, the depiction on the sketch conveys the number and type of injuries clearly. In thermal injuries or burn injuries which are quite common in India, amongst newly married females, due to reasons of dowry (elaborate gifts from bride's family as per the demand from the groom's family) the depiction of burns on the sketch is able to show the extent and pattern of burns. Extent of coronary occlusion means the amount of blockage of coronary arteries of the heart. For this an outline 2D sketch of coronaries of heart are used and places of block with extent of block is mentioned in percentage. This report then is collected by the police officer of the investigating police station and submitted to the court. The judge or the Magistrate in the court issues summons for the witnesses including the doctors and autopsy surgeons. These summons are hand delivered by the policeman. The summon informs the date on which one is expected in the court, the case trial number, the section of the penal code under which the case is registered and the name of the accused. The summon is always accompanied by its carbon copy. The receipt of the summon is taken by the police officer, on the copy of the summon, as evidence that the summon has been served. If the court is an out station court, we are relieved of our routine duties for the purpose of attending the court. Giving evidence in court for some is an inconvenient experience. After attending a few courts, getting to know the relevance of one's evidence and developing a style of depositing evidence a court evidence becomes a good mental exercise and informative and sometimes fulfilling or even thrilling at times.

Giving evidence in courts has technical aspect to it and equally important, to have a perspective and attitude for it. As postgraduate students, we accompanied the Faculty to courts, local or distant, when they went for their evidence. When we went to adjoining districts, the journey time would become an interactive time and we would get to share their experiences and outlook to various aspects of work. Working in Forensic Medicine means appearing in court to deposit evidence about 70 – 100 times in a year, doing about 200 – 300 autopsies a year and examining about 100 – 150 medico legal cases related to age estimation, injuries and sexual offences. There are thus, quite a number of times when we are giving evidence in two or more cases in a day.

Being a referral institute for autopsies from around Bhopal, there would be lots of difficult cases and decomposed bodies with good findings. It of course means lots of out station court evidences. These places usually include small towns or places which require one to travel through rural India. Till a few years back, it implied bad roads with slow and overcrowded buses. Now the roads are better over the years and often we travel by our own cars. Going to courts in smaller towns and semi rural places means looking at green fields, seeing people dressed traditionally and sometimes new experiences. The courtrooms are far from being glamorous and usually are housed in old buildings which are very poorly maintained. Only a very few places have court buildings which have been designed to be courts. In the courts, when we give evidence, it is recorded as examination-in-chief and then we are cross-examined by the lawyer of the defendant. As most of our routine work and curriculum is in English, we enter patient details, diagnosis and findings in English. The prescriptions, case sheets and medico-legal reports all are in English, but when we give evidence, we are expected to deposit our evidence in Hindi. This is quite a task the first few times and gradually eases out. Over the years, Forensic experts are the most frequent visitors to court from amongst the doctors. Hence, when a Forensic expert is submitting the deposition, the statement is recorded with minimal interference and proceeds with clarity, as they are conversant with the language to be used in court, the protocol and chronology of facts as they are to be deposited. There being few Forensic experts in the state, all have their own identity and reputation and most of the time the court realizes the effort we make to reach out-station courts and so they usually make effort to have our evidence submitted quickly. The courts are usually extremely considerate if a doctor comes to court, from a long distance and has the return journey shortly. In the past 20 years, except for a few stray incidences, sitting or waiting in court has never happened.

A lot of circumstances have improved in the past 10 years with road connections having improved remarkably, cutting travel time to half for some places. Now, one can practically take one's own private vehicle to all the places with perfect ease. The journeys are a pleasure. Staying in a city, visiting smaller towns around and traveling through the countryside, meeting people of the rural and semi-urban areas, watching their perspectives, way of living and attitudes, taking a look at their lifestyles and standard of living is refreshing and stimulating in its own way. The outlook of people in such places sometimes feels primitive, sometimes just different and hence thought provoking and at times, quite simply, inspiring. Their simple ways of living, contentment and connectedness with nature are traits worth emulating.

Depositing or giving evidence is a skill and with time, connecting to a case as a witness, promotes our insight as to how we can provide a particular direction to a case. It soon becomes like a jigsaw, a mind game or a strategy game when one tries to see the overview of the case. But to enjoy this experience, the prerequisite is the intention to understand why and how our evidence is taken as it is taken. Depositing our evidence is a science, a skill. Understanding the science and discovering the art makes the experience wholesome. It then never gets boring or mundane. It is like a mind exercise and with time one can perceive how we can, as an expert, contribute to clarifying the facts within our purview and related to the case, and how they can be harnessed more effectively. One also learns to answer strategically the questions by the advocate and help in avoiding misinterpretations by the court. One is not boggled and occupied simply about giving facts of the case known in a proper way and walking out without having to answer the questions of the cross-examination. When one has acquired somewhat the skill of this deposition, the nervousness and stress of appearing in court and replying the questions put up, do not trouble one at all. It becomes a privilege and pleasure to be able to intervene in cases and simplify our findings for purpose of being used in the court. Medical evidence is very significant in some cases and in absence of other evidences, can do what no one else can do for the case. Those are the occasions where the knowledge and its applicability when demonstrated convincingly, can turn things, move things or make them as explicit as they ought to be. To me, it is one of the most enjoyable aspects of the job and something which never gets boring or monotonous. There is only one golden rule after one has understood the procedure of court evidence to harness that enjoyment – be patient always. Never be in a hurry to finish a case, to leave the court or to make a quick exit from questions and cross questions. There are occasions the court is not held, for which one has traveled long distance or has gone repeatedly, but never let such shortcomings deter you from the ultimate purpose. The autopsy, the knowledge of facts and their interpretations, the written reports and documents all serve one single purpose. The presentation and understanding by the court in those few minutes may give meaning to the whole work behind it. An opportunity lost then could make the whole difference between work well done and a defeated purpose. We do sometimes contemplate later how we could have improved the understanding and outcome in a case, but then it is sometimes too late. One needs to be patient, attentive, calm, logical and sometimes even assertive or enthusiastic. It takes time and experience coupled with desire to understand, keen interest and observation to understand the whole mechanism, line of inquiry, possible grey areas which are likely to be explored and exploited.

Medical field sometimes appears only partly technical with all its unpredictability and dominant human elements. It moves by probabilities and exceptions both. In medicine, we are taught common symptoms of an ailment, their causes and then the variations possible in their number and extent which may appear in an individual. We are then taught to put a certain degree of reliance on a particular conglomerate or set of signs. There are investigations which are specific to a particular disease or condition and some which are common to a group of conditions. Law on the other hand, goes by a fixed set of penal codes, looks at well-established and proven evidences only, accepting as evidence all that is reasonable and beyond a certain degree of doubt/certainty. Forensic Medicine is a bridge between the two. We understand admissibility of evidence and its objectivity better than other medical personnel and are able to explain the medical and Medicolegal terminology and its implications better to the court. As for example, the exact duration of disease or injury may not be possible to be stated, but minimum duration beyond reasonable doubt can be conveyed. The extent or type of injury which places it legally as simple or grievous may become a dilemma either due to lack of information or the injury coming into the grey area between the two categories. Here, the potential of injury in causing harm or complications may be quantified and explained with examples and citations from books easing the matter for the court and helping to steer the case on the right course. Sometimes, when a person has been hospitalized after sustaining the injury and succumbs to the injury, it is a common practice to shift blame from the person accused of having caused the injury to the doctor on grounds that the services provided were inadequate, inappropriate or negligent. Then the dilemma of assigning the degree of blame or onus of responsibility on either or both is raised. A person dying of a disease in police custody could also face a similar situation. When a person is in police custody and falls ill, he is provided medical services.

If he still deteriorates or dies, the onus of responsibility has to be fixed, either on the medical services or the police in whose custody the deceased was and whose responsibility it was to provide adequate care to the detained.

Court evidences outside Bhopal to adjacent areas, mainly in Madhya Pradesh, motivated me to drive on highways. It was something which I thought was quite adventurous but at the same time apprehended as something very difficult or demanding. With friends and family forever telling me the dangers of driving on a highway, there was one person who knew that highway driving and I would get along really well and that it was not at all like the invincible art it was made out to be, that it wasn't something which was impossible, rather something right there within reach – ready to be grasped and enjoyed! That was my boss who I often think can see through me like glass and read my heart and mind like a book. He voiced my fears before I did very often and was quicker than me in dismissing any illogical explanations and mind-blocks. He would often hand me the wheel of his car on a highway when we accompanied him for his court evidences as students. I admire the way he let me taste the fun of highway driving and then coaxed me into doing it. It opened a whole new vista of fun and journey for courts at distant places became something to look forward to. Driving on a highway is a 'high' in itself and to give it the name of job or duty made me feel guilty, it was so much fun!

One such outstation court I had been to recently exemplifies it clearly. I had a court evidence at Biaora, Rajgarh, about 130 kms from Bhopal. I have been to this place several times but mostly in the car. This time for some reason the car was not available and I thought of trying the bus ride. The car takes about one and half to two hours and so I presumed the bus would take about two and half hours. When I saw the bus for Biaora it was literally filled to capacity and the next bus an hour away. The conductor confirmed whether I wanted to board the bus about to leave and on affirmation, he asked me to be seated. Although the bus was full he asked me not to worry and that he would ensure the journey to be comfortable. On entering the bus, he just asked loudly to the people sitting in the last row that they better make place for a lady passenger. The young men, somewhat grudgingly shrunk and created the space. They were freshly appointed teachers in a school in Biaora. While talking to them I realized that they were interested in seeing an autopsy and in knowing what my work involves and the whole concept of a court evidence. They also realized that I must reach in a time frame to complete my work, so they began to worry about me getting late. The bus reached Biaora at about 2 pm. When I reached the court, I realized that the court was to be held in Rajgarh, about 25 kms from the place I had reached, which would take me another half an hour. They had specified Rajgarh (Biaora) only to convey that this is the particular Rajgarh and not either of the other two Rajgarh(s). A lawyer at the court offered a ride on his motor bike and dropped me to the bus stand and then I reached Rajgarh. I rushed to the court, gave evidence and rushed back. The bus in which I was now seated was crowded and I could smell the country liquor around me. In Biaora, I had to change the bus and now I was sitting with a goat next to me, a possibility which was unheard and unseen even in my nightmares. I was finally home at about 8 pm. A journey which should have been four hours took nine hours! But those extra five hours gave me a glimpse of what many people go through, their lives and attitudes and a memorable experience of travelling with the goat. To this day I remember the episode as strange and funny. It was remarkable how the co-passengers were comfortable with the goat and accepted it as just another co- passenger.

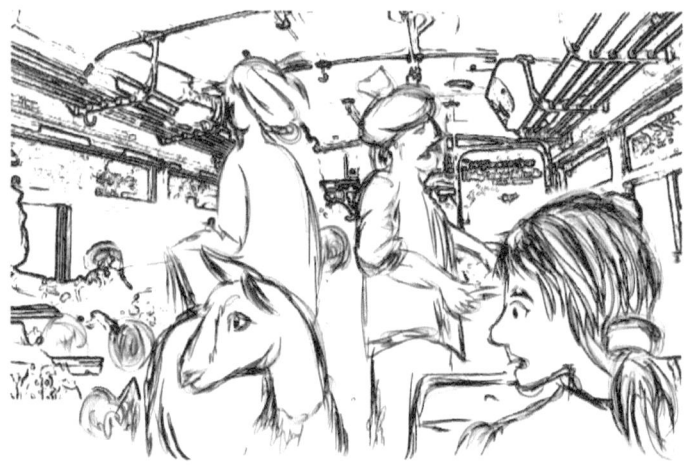

Somewhere around 2001, I received a summon from the court of Lateri. Apprehension to travel to Lateri was substantial for it was not well connected. The effort to find the appropriate conveyance / transport means had started a week earlier. Lateri is a village of district Vidisha close to Bhopal, but with no Railway Station and does not have a good connection by road. To be more explicit, there were no roads for quite a long distance around it. One heard of stories how people travelling to Lateri with vehicles had to stop to make way for themselves by removing the big boulders/stones in their way. Here is what I wrote then after attending a court there.

There are many experiences of travelling for court evidences in areas where there were either no roads or really bad roads in the late 90s and even early part of this century. One of the places which was difficult to reach from Bhopal by road or train was Lateri. There were three buses to Lateri, one leaving at 8:25 am, the other at 10:15 am and the third at 11:15 am. Each of them would take about 4 to 4 and half hours for these 115 kms! It was indeed a desperate attempt to catch the morning bus and being seated in that bus itself made one feel victorious. The roads were bad, to say the least. There was practically no road. Every time the bus stopped and this happened whenever anyone wanted to board the bus on the way, there would be a cloud of mud, stark red mud. There were tall prickly shrubs along the way hitting the people's faces and arms who were sitting near the window, unless they deliberately pulled themselves away from the window. Many a times one would marvel at the driver's instinct of knowing exactly where to go even without a road. The state of the buses explained the roads really. The seats were hard, without enough cushioning, the windows with broken or semi broken glasses, their metal frames shaking and creating a jarring loud noise. Shock absorbers were perhaps alien to the bus and if one did not hold the metal bar on the back rest of the seat in front of us, we could be thrown high enough to hit the roof with our heads.

The map of Madhya Pradesh shows National and State Highways and other roads too. The day before leaving I was peering into a map and brooding over the status of road, and could not see a road directly between Shamshabad and Lateri (remember this is the era before the age of google maps). As it turned out, there was no road, but the buses were running on this track, ignoring the absence of road.

After crossing the relatively easy 45 kms, the bus stopped at the crossing of Shamshabad. I needed to use a toilet then. The conductor told me where the toilet was, which was about 100 m from the crossing. He suggested an option whereby I could spend about 10-15 min at the crossing and have tea and snacks available. The bus would go into the town of Shamshabad, drop and collect passengers and then come back to this crossing to proceed for Lateri. It seemed like a good offer except for a slightly insecure feeling of being stranded at this crossing for 15 min. It of course would spare me the rocking movement and vibrations for 15 min. So, I responded affirmatively, trusting him spontaneously. Looking at the toilet, getting nauseated was the only response. It was an unroofed small structure, with space for a couple of toilets adjacent to each other. Inside, there was hardly any clean space to keep one's foot, even if one had decided to use it. There was so much of shit, mud and bad smell that it was unthinkable to use the toilet. All along the journey there was absolutely no toilet anywhere and the only option to go for toilet was on the roadside.

Further along the way, there came small rivers, lakes, forests and small villages and I wondered each time whether the bus would be able to go further or would get stuck right there. But the driver very confidently, each time, almost with deft certainty, put the bus through the uneven terrain knowing that it would like all previous days, pass through. He could decide to go, which way to go, in which direction, even when there was no way in sight anywhere. It looked amazing; it felt risky and took its toll on the passengers physically with all the big jolts, sudden turns, rough terrain and undaunting driving skills!

At one time, an old woman sat beside me. I casually remarked that the roads are awful, she thought for a while and said that this was hardly a problem compared to the problem which arises in rainy weather when the road gets blocked. The people in that region cannot be stopped by the absence of roads. They will stop only when they simply cannot go. As I sat on my window seat munching the fruits I was carrying with me, I wondered what made people continue to live in such areas, far from active social life, in isolated and quiet pockets. The only sound of developed life they hear is the sound of the vehicle passing by. Children actually gather around and stare at the bus and its passengers, whenever it seems to pass by. But then again, it seems that these are the very people who know what it means to have a simple living. They know exactly that basic food, minimal clothing and shelter is all that is really needed to survive. The people of the villages with their typical accent and way of dressing were very interesting; their outlook and grit and the undeterred stamina to face the hardships was all quite impressive. Yet it feels very guilty to see them living in this state decades after being a democracy.

What was also very touching at the end of the day was when I was reaching back Bhopal at about 6 pm, my teacher and boss, came to pick me from the bus stand! He was remembering the time he had been to Lateri. He realised what I must have gone through and how I might be feeling at the end of the day. We compared notes. Nothing much had changed really. We now shared a common memory, journey to the court rather than the court evidence itself!

Over last two decades I have noticed that when a doctor is summoned to appear in court even as an expert witness, he or she has lot of apprehensions. Most of these apprehensions are not worth nurturing. If the doctor has been involved with treatment, he must just keep in mind that the court only wants to the details of the treatment and the type of injury in a case of trauma. The court in no way intends to harass or question a doctor's competence. The courts usually respect a doctor's skill and time and try to bring to minimum the time spent by the doctor in court. Anything overlooked by the doctor in the best interest of the patient, while focused on the treatment, could be taken considerately by the court, when justified well. It would only be recommended for the doctor to be confident, maintain serious demeanour and to never over opinionate. The doctor must only keep in mind that it is his duty to help law find truth and understand from clinical point of view what exactly happened and how things progressed.

Special cases

There are routine cases and there are special cases, and the distinction is an after thought. A routine case sometimes holds more lessons and attracts more interest than a special case. Routine autopsy cases include road traffic accidents, hanging, poisoning and burn cases. I share excerpts from a few cases here, each for a special reason and hope that they convey some information of interest.

Case number 1

In a particular geographical region, people show preference to use of a particular poison over all others either for reasons of availability or cost. Sometimes a particular poison in a region gets fame (or ill fame) for its certainty of action and desired end result, literally. Most common poisoning cases seen at autopsy in Central region of India include those due to consumption of organophosphates (a group of insecticides) and Aluminum phosphide (rodenticide). Then there are others relatively less often used and then some used extremely rarely. It is interesting how we reach the diagnosis of a particular poison in a case of poisoning at autopsy. A case could exemplify it better.

A young male about 30 years of age was found dead at his work place around 11am. He worked in a pharmaceutical company as a Scientist. In the mortuary we could not find any external signs of injury and the congestion (reddening) of his face was prominent. At autopsy, internally there were no grossly apparent findings related to any disease or trauma. Inner lining of stomach was markedly congested and there was a peculiar odour I had not smelt earlier. On completion of autopsy, the cause of death was written as poisoning and the samples of organs were given in the Toxicology laboratory of the department for chemical analysis. When such a sample reaches a toxicologist, he or she faces the dilemma of identifying the poison. Of all the poisons it can be, to identify a specific one is a major issue. It requires some clues, some suspicions, which can be confirmed or refuted. With limited sample size, interacting with the forensic pathologist is the best strategy, to get a clue. As forensic pathologist, we want to know the details of the poison. This interdependence followed by communication holds the key most often in a case of poisoning. In this particular case when I met the Chemical Examiner the next day on my way to the Mortuary, he asked me about the findings. When I told him about the thick layer of congestion on gastric mucosa (lining of stomach), dark in colour and with a peculiar odour, he thought and suspected a few compounds. I could not describe the odour to him at all and then he had another bright idea. He got a few chemicals in test tubes lined up and asked me to smell them. This was not the smell and I began to wonder whether this would work. I waited a while before smelling the next test tube with a different chemical. This time I could not believe it. This was exactly the same odour I had smelt. The toxicologist then suggested whether the odour resembled that of bitter almonds. When he mentioned it, I realised that it did in a very strong and exaggerated way! He then told me that the chemical I had found similar in smell to the sample in question, was cyanide. Chemical analysis confirmed it. It was my absolute first acquaintance with a case of cyanide poisoning and I had participated in its discovery. Then came the role of investigating agency to establish where the cyanide could have come from. The police revisited the place where the body was found, and realised that he did have access to cyanide in the laboratory he worked.

Impression: This case brings out the importance of interaction between a Forensic Pathologist and the toxicologist in a case of suspected poisoning.

Case number 2

This particular case happened more than ten years ago, in August 2005.

Dead body of a 5 year old female child was brought for autopsy. A salwar (Indian pants for women tied by a string around the waist when worn) was tied around neck. The deceased belonged to a home in the slums in the centre of the city. Dileep, aged about 35 years who lived in the same locality, was reported to have taken the girl with him. He took her to Bagh Mugalia area, about 20 kms away in the outskirts of the city, in the fields, where he raped and killed her. The body was recovered from the fields when somebody reported a dead body there. For Dileep, it was his fourth crime. About 20 years ago, he had been charged with offence of sexual assault on a girl aged about 6-8 years and was convicted for 7 years. On completing the term of his punishment, he again sexually assaulted a girl aged about 4-5 years. This time he was awarded punishment for 3 years. On returning after completing the term of his second imprisonment, he again in a few months, committed the crime on his sister-in-law's daughter aged about 4 years. Being related to the accused and partly due to social pressures, the aggrieved and the accused opted for an out of court settlement. The accused some time later, again attempted to commit the same crime on a girl aged about 6 years, but the girl somehow managed to escape and the matter was not pursued any further. This time, it was perhaps the 4th time that this act was repeated, the neighbours and residents of the area were quite agitated and got the accused arrested.

The girl on examination had a bruise on right side of her forehead, about 1.5 × 2 cm size and had multiple abrasions and bruises on the lower back in an a area 17.5 × 15 cm, vertical. Salwar tied around the neck had a double fixed knot on both the sides. Underneath was the mark on neck (called ligature mark) and bruise on left outer aspect in the front with underlying muscles bruised. Skin had been pinched between folds of the cloth. The external genitalia showed a wound with bruise on the lower part of labia majora and minora. The hymen was also torn. Underlying muscles were exposed and there was oozing of blood. There was also abrasion and bruise on upper outer side of left thigh. These findings are associated with violent sexual assault. The cause of death was asphyxia of strangulation. The signs of violent sexual assault were reported. At autopsy, injuries and other findings are sometimes so clear and self explanatory, that the presence of crime, the volume of force used, the intention and the place of crime all are explained or verified. The autopsy surgeons in such cases should be able to objectively observe and record these findings and secure photographic evidence or show injuries on a sketch diagram.

Judgement of the case was given a year and half later by the Session Judge of Bhopal. The judgement made headlines because the case was well worked up on, a serial offender was the accused and the crime of child abuse was continually repeated. The judge announced death sentence for he felt that no punishment less than capital punishment would suffice. It was one of the first cases in Bhopal where the accused was awarded death sentence. Death sentence in India is given by hanging. Capital punishment when given by session (highest district) court, is to be confirmed by high court of the state to be executed. The infrastructure for hanging is not available in all district courts. Death sentence overall, in India is quite infrequent. It is usual for death sentence to be changed to life imprisonment by the appellate courts. The facility to execute hanging does not exist in Bhopal. Hence, the accused was then postulated to be sent to either Indore or Gwalior to be hanged.

Impression: A detailed work up and clear presentation in court makes it easy for the judge to decide the punishment to be awarded.

Case number 3

Another case of 2006 is of a 65 year old man who lived with his four sons at Pachore, a village near Narsinghgarh in Rajgarh district. He complained of chest pain on right lateral aspect of chest, seemingly in the ribs. He was taken to a doctor by one of his sons. The doctor administered an injection on right upper arm, gave some medication and sent him home. The next day the man complained of pain in his right upper limb. His family members convinced him that the pain must be due to the injection and that it would go in a day or two. The next day he noticed swelling of his right upper limb and some stiffness. The doctor, on request, came home to examine the old man. He now gave some ointment to be applied on the limb and assured them that it would be fine. But the condition continued to deteriorate. So they now took him to a bigger hospital in Biaora. Here the doctor realized that the patient had gangrene and would require expert care. He was referred to a higher centre, a tertiary level government hospital at Bhopal. He reached Bhopal but died in a few hours.

On autopsy, signs of gangrene were evident. The right upper limb was swollen, dark and crepitant. Vertical incisions on medial aspect of right arm were present and a long incision on back of the right arm on inner side 4 cm below the armpit up to 6 cm above wrist was present and muscles exposed. Muscles were soft, dark and crepitant and foul smelling pus present at places. Blisters were seen on the skin at places. Venesection was done in the left arm above the elbow and ointment was present over the right upper limb.

The doctor at Pachore, who had given the injection was trained in Homeopathic system of medicine and legally not entitled to give any Allopathic medicine. A registration in Homeopathic Medical Council gives him the right to prescribe homeopathic drugs and treatment, but he is legally barred to prescribe in any other pathy. When the case developed gas gangrene as a result of his injection, he could either not diagnose it or could not give proper treatment or refer the case to a higher centre in time and thus was charged under section 304 A IPC. A person is charged under this section of Indian Penal Code (IPC) for rash, negligent act. His lawyer tried to shift blame to the consecutive clinician who had seen the case. The consecutive clinician had exercised due care and skill in giving linear incisions on the right upper limb, diagnosing it as gas gangrene and advising to shift the case to a tertiary care centre was not considered guilty by the court.

Impression: Reconstruction of the case and correlation of the history with the findings can make the inquest easier.

Case number 4

Sometimes one gets to know the most phenomenal real life stories during autopsy. The case being described is one of those. This was 2004 and a case with burns as the cause of death was brought for autopsy. The case was that of a Kinnar (eunuch), with name on the requisition written as Kinnar Archana, wife of Arjun, aged 20 years. To know more about the case, we talked to Arjun. He was about 25 years old, in love with the Kinnar and had been living with 'her' for about 2 years. The memories of these two years of cohabitation were held fondly by Arjun as blissful and happy. When she sustained burns, he took her for treatment to the District hospital in Biaora, where they lived. When her condition did not improve, she was referred to Bhopal and she died 2 days later. She had about 80-90% burns. There were no external genitalia and only remains of what seemed to be prostatic tissue by its location and firmness and remains of vas deferens, the spermatic cord as internal genitalia. A linear healed scar was present over the pubic region, which remained as the only evidence of the surgery she had undertaken about 2 months back to get the remains of the external genitalia removed, a surgery which cost her about Rs.25,000/=. The surgery was voluntarily opted for by the couple so that Archana could feel and be a little more 'female.' Now Arjun took on himself to perform all the burial rights. The marriage (acceptable or unacceptable), its completeness or incompleteness, legal sanction, Archana being a Muslim and Arjun being a Hindu, nothing had any deterrent effect on his affection for her or their bondage. That he was so much in love that he did not realize that he is not her husband legally, but could not care less. He was the only attendant with her and not once did he flinch from admitting any part of his story, that he was going through the grueling exercise of handling a Medicolegal case single-handedly and yet respecting her religious feelings, was worth appreciation. Archana, he clarified, was a Muslim and was called "Aanchal" and was re-named by him as Archana on cohabitation. Now that she was dead, he was going to bury her as is done in Muslim tradition, as opposed to Hindus, who are cremated (burnt on a pyre). This was his final respect to her spirituality and religion, which he was doing with no hesitation and no conflicts. A eunuch learnt for 'herself' and taught a person the principle of love, marriage, religion and justice in a manner unknown to many usual couples. Yet, these are the people who have to fight for their identity, rights and status. Husbands handle burnt infected bodies of their wives, with lot of reluctance, and this person, shaken and yet so much in love, they could have lived happily all their lives, incomplete as they were, but death did part them. Yes, it is very rare to see love after death of a person and it can be seen very easily, whenever it is there. Such deaths make you think a lot about why(s) of life and its meaning and these faces do not get wiped out from the mind. I wonder if it all leads to some psychological occupational hazard, because it sometimes makes me think why am I to witness end of such lives rather than the happy lives while they last, and at other times I feel thankful that at least I got to know that the human instinct lives and is not dead.

Impression: A routine appearing case can become interesting if history of the case is explored. Detailed examination is important in every case.

Case number 5

A beautiful day in November 2004, was a regular working day with autopsies, practical undergraduate demonstration and a meeting-to-attend type of day. I was wondering why I could not be outdoors and photographing. Almost as an answer to it, there was a call from Deputy Inspector General of Police stating that a dead body was found at Budhni, about 80 kms from Bhopal at the banks of river Narmada, which is likely to be the one thrown after murder, about 7 days back from the bridge over the Narmada. The next day was election day all over the state and because this case was known to have aroused fury of the people earlier, they wanted the autopsy to be done the same day to prevent any law and order problem on the election day. Repair of railway line too was going on near Budhni and so traffic load on the highway had also increased, as only one lane was being used. Getting the dead body from the site that it was present and bringing it to the mortuary of Bhopal would not have been possible till 5pm, so it was requested that the autopsy surgeons reach the site and conduct the autopsy there. I accompanied Dr Badkur and we left our workplace at 1:45 pm. We were accompanied by the investigating officer of the case, the two accused (handcuffed), two constables and the driver. The accused were South Indians, graduates, running small independent business of a travel agency and a STD/ PCO telephone booth. They both had previous elaborate criminal record, were bachelors and quite open to informing details of the sequence of events. Over time they were seasoned to realize that if they told all the details to police there would not be any physical assault and getting free is a matter to be decided by the court, which somehow was not reason enough to be worried. They described how a group of about 4 friends would not get along with this group of 4 people and so there were occasional clashes. Both groups of people were fond of consuming alcoholic drinks which they did almost on a regular basis. This particular night of 12thNov, they had their drinks and decided to have fun with the other group by having a collision with them. The accident they believed would give the some injuries and it would be some time before they recoup their original self again. Under the influence of alcohol they did feel a little lost with their train of thoughts and actions. The plan was executed as planned and after the accident they thought it was enough trouble and injuries and so they decide to drop them at the nearby hospital. While doing so the two victims in the vehicle died. They then decided to throw one of them, a 20 year old man who was recently married, off the bridge into the Narmada river. The other body, they dropped at another place Betul. This body was autopsied at Betul. The accused travelling with us insisted that all they intended was a mere accident and unfortunately it terminated as death. They also admitted in the informal conversation during the journey that if they had not consumed alcohol, perhaps they would not have done such an act. While going on the way, we almost got caught up in the traffic jam like situation with repair of the railway line going on over the State Highway road with large number of trucks (lorries) moving over it in that region. We reached the Narmada bridge, in about two hours by 3:45pm, a place we should have reached in about an hour. We had to walk down from the bridge and then along one of the banks and reach where the body was found. The full, bounding Narmada, its quietness and soft rumbling squishy sound created a silent and austere feel. The sandy bank was soon replaced by black soil bank and the expanse of the river and its stillness made one contemplate about petty reasons for crime and throwing of the body into the holy river. Narmada considered a holy river, probably second only to the Ganga in terms of religious reverence it receives. After nearly a kilometer walk, we reached the place where dead skeletal remains had been brought up to the bushes. A few bones were still scattered around. The skull attached to the vertebrae and ribs, hip bones and femur was found in one piece. The lower jaw, pieces of right arm and forearm bones, right leg bones, left collarbone and scapula together were found scattered around the body a little scattered. They were all brought together and examined. The bones were all of the same individual, of male aged about 25 years. The clothes and a black thread with a metallic pendant identified as worn by the deceased were also recovered from the river. It is amazing how all the evidence could be recovered from the riverside and it helped to substantiate the crime committed nearly 7 days ago. The skull contained liquefied remains of brain and only at few places remains of ligaments were still present. Fractures of right zygomatic arch and maxillary sinus, right 3rd, 4th and 5th ribs at paravertebral regions, L3,4,5 and S1,2,3 vertebrae were fractured. These fractures were ante-mortem. Bones also showed gnawing effect by animals at their ends mainly. Having completed the examination at about 5:30pm, it was thought proper to preserve the skull along with mandible for superimposition should the question of identity be raised later. It was satisfying to note that the autopsy had finished just in time when it was beginning to get dark. A few persons of the media had also come and a crowd of about 50 to 60 people were silent observers of the whole process. The bony remains were burnt at the banks of Narmada with a short condolence ceremony organized by the Superintendent of Police.

A visit to the spot helps to get inputs from many people and helps to understand the case better.

A year and two months later, on 2nd Jan 2006, I was summoned as witness to attend the court for this case. The four accused were represented by their lawyers, all of them well-known criminal lawyers. The doctor from Betul who had performed the autopsy was being cross-examined and when he finished, I was asked to deposit my evidence. One of the advocates asked whether the fractures could be due to accidental, suicidal or homicidal fall. It was practically not possible to be certain of any manner or intent by merely the autopsy findings. Considering the circumstantial evidence, it is obviously homicidal but there would be lot of suggestions and arments for refusal of this theory on grounds of lack of conclusive evidence or perhaps using discretion and proceeding by exclusion, an opinion may emerge with reasonable certainty. One of the advocates wanted to confirm whether the remains were close to the railway bridge or the road bridge and yet another was trying to ascertain when the person got identified before, after or during the autopsy.

Impression: A spot examination can sometimes reveal lot more information than when the body is examined in the Mortuary.

Case number 6

The military box in the Goa express was unattended for quite some time, so it was brought down at Bhopal station and opened. It contained dead body of a relatively old man in a partly decomposed stage. It was then sent for post-mortem examination. The box was a military box abandoned in the train and contained dead body of a relatively old unknown person, in moderate stage of decomposition with shoe laces tied around the neck. All this made it sound like an unusual challenge.

The deceased wore a dhoti (cloth tied around waist) secured in the front by two knots, in a typical 'Marathi' (people belonging to Maharashtra region of the country) way. He was also wearing a vest, had baldness appearing in the vault region, with about 30% grey hair among the rim of hair around the head. The skin had started peeling. The shoe lace was tied around the neck with a fixed knot on the front of the neck on right side. On removing this lace according to the autopsy protocol, there was a well-defined, grooved, ligature mark (as it is called) reflecting the pattern of the lace. On giving a cut over the mark, there was a pale, white glistening appearance under the mark and marginal ecchymosis (bruising on the margin of the mark) well marked. The internal organs were soft and spleen was in liquefying stage. The cause of death was strangulation, manner of death homicidal and duration of death 2 to 3 days before the post-mortem examination. Identification points were noted and photographs taken. The person was identified later by the police and the history with sequence of events somewhat placed together.

A soldier in the army lived close to Ahmednagar, a small town in Maharashtra with his brother, parents and wife. Army required him to be away from home for long duration. His wife developed liking for his brother in the circumstances. When the parents learnt of this, they asked their son and daughter-in-law to refrain from such acts and that it was highly unethical. When the the son in the army came home on holiday, before the parents could say anything, the wife complained to her husband that she was being accused falsely of infidelity by her in-laws and that she was mentally tortured on that account. The husband accepted the wife's version of events and was enraged at his parent's and sister's behaviour, who lived close by. One evening, he killed his parents and sister and put their bodies in a box. He then hired a van, loaded the trunks in the van and brought them to Ahmednagar railway station. His wife and brother also helped in disposal of these dead bodies. The trunks were then loaded on separate trains and they returned back home. The trunk which contained the dead body of his father was loaded in Goa express and a woman noticed the man keeping such a big trunk. When the train reached Bhopal station, nobody claimed the trunk. The trunk by its size and being unclaimed, aroused the interest of the other passengers. Then someone noticed dark coloured, foul-smelling fluid coming out from the trunk, when the railway police came in and intervened. They opened the trunk and found the dead body inside. The woman who was closely watching the person loading the trunk on the trunk furnished the details required by the police and the description of the person too. She was the prime witness in the case who could by her memory later identify the accused too. Her description of the person also fitted exactly the person himself. A saree in the trunk further helped in identification, as it was gifted to the wife of the victim by her sister-in-law and was of a particular brand by which the origin could be traced.

Two years later, I was summoned to the court of Ahmednagar, 13 hours of train journey from Bhopal. It was an overnight journey, with evidence in the court scheduled in the morning. The return journey would be the next night. The court of a different state raised some anxiety for each state has its own way of working. At Ahmednagar in Maharashtra state, the proceedings of the court were recorded in either Marathi or English as opposed to Hindi in Madhya Pradesh.

The court was pleased to see an autopsy report more detailed than their usual one, accompanied by photographs to illustrate and explain the findings better. I was adviced by my teacher and boss Dr Dubey to take the photographs along as it might serve to simplify an explanation and show the findings clearly. I was cross examined on several issues some of which were trivial, but all along I noticed that the judge was absorbing all the information with lot of sensibility and soon the picture was crystal clear in his mind. I was left with no doubt that the things were taken in the expected spirit and with the required understanding. The court evidence took about one and half hours but was worth all the effort, as this was a case where there were no eyewitnesses, but circumstantial evidence and inquest were to get credit for sorting out the case.

Impression: Skill and effort of autopsy sometimes have no substitute.

Case number 7

A one and half year old girl was brought for autopsy examination. She was a Nepali in origin. Her parents were part of a group of people who would come to India from Nepal every winter, sell their hand knitted woolens through the temporary shops and return home having sold their goods. This visit would stretch commonly to 3 or 4 months when they went back with all they had earned. During this time, they would work all day leaving their daughter at home with a 10 year old Nepali boy. One particular day, two young men who were aware of this routine and expected to find reasonable amount of money at home, came with plan to extort it with only the boy around at that time. They found some money and expecting more, continued to explore. The 10 year old boy, who had been entrusted with looking after the small child, tried to stop them. A scuffle followed, when the two intruders picked the small child and dropped her on the hard stony ground from a height of about 4 feet. The child sustained head injuries and died a few hours later. On autopsy there was contusion on the scalp and substantial intracranial haemorrhage which was the cause of death. The summon for the court evidence came about 6 months after the autopsy. On cross examination several issues were raised, some of which seemed distinctly irrelevant. I was asked whether the eyes being open or close was related to intracranial haemorrhages, what I meant by medial or inner surface and temporal surface or outer surface of brain and for how long the child might have survived after sustaining the injuries. Survival time suggested by history was about 18 hours, which was consistent with the autopsy findings. The defence lawyer then sought opinion whether this type of head injury could be attributed to the fall from the bed and hence should the manner of death be considered as accidental or as homicidal by dropping from a height. The circumstantial evidence which were taken into account to analyse the manner of death included the type of floor of the house and the possible heights from which the fall could have taken place. The floor had rectangular slabs of stone and the height of the bed was about 2 feet. The contusion and the intracranial haemorrhage seemed to indicate a forceful throw on the ground. The skull in the first 2-3 years, is single layered and elastic as compared to that of bigger children and adults, where it is three layered. Hence the skull in early years does not fracture easily, rather bends inwards easily and gets indented. The intracranial haemorrhage in such cases becomes a good indicator of the force sustained. The magnitude of the injury in this case did not coincide with an accidental fall from the bed and rather seemed more appropriate for a forceful fall from a height of about 4-5 feet. Besides being winter season at this time of the year, the baby being well wrapped in warm clothes had been admitted by the accused and chances of sustaining injuries by a gentle fall were further reduced.

Impression: A sound judgement based on experience can sometimes provide good evidence.

Case number 8

Autopsy on a 20 year old male was done in August 2000. There was a healed linear scar on left ear, the scar extending beyond the ear posteriorly on the mastoid bone. The length of the scar was 10cms. A yellow foul smelling discharge of pus was also seen in the left ear. On removing the scalp, a transverse fracture, 1.5 cm long was seen on the mastoid bone with sharp bony edge directed inwards. This bony projection was felt in the petrous part of temporal bone, which is seen on removing the brain. There was surrounding blackish discolouration of necrosis. Dura was torn and a large intracerebral temporal pus was seen, extending on the base and the superior surface of the brain. A thick covering what we call a capsule, was also beginning to form around the pus and there was sloughing of brain in the temporal lobe.

There was history of an argument of the deceased with his brother over inheritance regarding a property, which continued to escalate to the extent that his brother hit him with an axe. On healing of this outer wound, the deceased had left for home against precautionary medical advice in about 10 -15 days after the injury was inflicted. About a month later he developed headache and other neurological symptoms. He reported to the hospital, but died within 24 hours. I was summoned to court three years later, in 2003 to a place called Sohagpur about 128 kilometres from my place when the post-mortem report of this case was found to be missing by the court. Again, in July 2004, I was issued a warrant to attend this case and instructed to come with a copy of the post mortem report. Sohagpur is about 3 hours away from Bhopal, and road was under construction at a few places and at some places in terrible shape. It was a rainy day which made the condition of the road worse. I had set out in the car at 9.30 am and reached the court at 12.30pm. I was informed that the Additional session judge was on half day casual leave and would come to court at 2.30pm. I visited an acquaintance in Sohagpur and came back to court at 2.30pm. Now the judge was back but he got involved in writing a judgement and then taking witnesses to other cases. So, it was a long wait upto 4.15 pm. Then I was called for evidence which was followed by cross-examination. I was questioned as to why I was calling the injury head injury, when the injury was over the ear and not in the head. It took quite an effort and patience to convince the court how ear and its skeleton were part of the head itself and thus injury was rightfully described as head injury. Then the process of abscess formation and its capsulation beginning to occur placed the minimum duration of injury to be 10 to 15 days. The cause of death was established to be head injury and its complications. Clinical details of the quality of treatment and better patient compliance would be further debated by the clinician and the evidence from the attendants of the patient. After a 45 minutes session of evidence and cross examination, I started for home at about 5pm. I reached Bhopal at about 8.30pm.

Impression: Court evidence and presentation in the court can sometimes explain more than a document.

CRITICAL ANALYSIS OF THE SUBJECT AND FUTURE DIRECTIONS

Routine technology or basic facility which should be available in Mortuary is not available at most places in the country. Any and all kinds of table are used as autopsy table. Regular water supply in the mortuaries does not exist in many. Comparatively, the mortuaries attached to government medical colleges are a step better. It is mandatory for a medical college to have a mortuary of a particular size. Qualified and trained mortuary technicians working in a mortuary is a rarity.

The ventilation in the mortuary, drainage of wastes or effluents from the mortuary after treating them to make them harmless, use of required kind of autopsy table are the basics required in any working mortuary, but are available in only a few elite institutions. An oscillating electric saw is ideally required to open the skull in autopsy in every autopsy case. As the saw is not available, skull is most commonly opened by hammer and chisel, a technique known to have many disadvantages. The hand held instruments required for autopsy are not available in many mortuaries. Routine supplies required for autopsy work like the gloves, cotton, suture material (thread for stitching the body after completion of autopsy), bottles for preservation of blood or tissue samples from autopsy, preservative chemicals and solutions, glass slides, etc are not available at many places. Many doctors at primary and community health centres are not trained in autopsy work, but have to regularly conduct autopsies. It is indeed surprising that in spite of these circumstances, all cases of homicide, trauma and decomposed bodies are autopsied and investigation continues based on the findings of these autopsy reports.

Most medical college mortuaries are overburdened with autopsies. In medical colleges, a Forensic medicine person who does autopsies is also involved in cases of clinical forensic medicine which includes cases related to age estimation and giving expert opinion in referred cases of sexual assault and trauma. Undergraduate and / or postgraduate courses in medical colleges also demand Forensic medicine person to take lectures and practical demonstrations, in addition to academic activities like seminars and presentations. In a teaching institute, it is mandatory to be involved in conducting examinations and in research projects and having results of research published. All these mandatory activities along with court evidences locally and beyond, depending which place the deceased belong to or where the case is registered are handled by Forensic persons.

More trained people need to be available and appointed for autopsy work to ensure quality autopsy work. Training in histopathology also needs to be upgraded for post graduates in Forensic medicine.

Autopsy service and related investigations are provided free of cost in India. It thus consumes money but does not generate any clinical advantage. The importance and the implications of a well performed autopsy are also not known to many. It could be the answer to doubts and suspicions regarding death of a close family member or friend or clarify the cause of a mysterious sudden death. Hence often people resist having an autopsy conducted on family members or close friends.

Private medical colleges have autopsies get the necessary permissions to conduct autopsy at their campus because it is a necessity to demonstrate autopsies to undergraduate students.

The ideal Mortuary is required to have a minimum size and other associated facilities like minimum instruments, lighting, water and proper ventilation or provision of personal protective equipment. Government run mortuaries are not much different either which need to be updated with current infection control recommendations.

Only few persons in few places are able to keep themselves updated and are able to carry on the important scientific work with inevitable legal implications in a satisfactory way.

Using videos for demonstration of court procedures to undergraduates could be very helpful. The short films or video clips could be a great learning tool.

Data of deaths or crime or judgements in India are not available or accessible. They do not get compiled or integrated which could perhaps provide an insight into crime, standard of medical care and death certification.

The time between autopsy and court evidence related to it is sometimes within a year but sometimes several years.

Future directions:

Forensic Medicine subject has lot more in the future for there is so much to do and so much to change. It requires more research activity to be incorporated as routine activity. There are less people involved in research and less research being directed to solving practical challenges. Estimation of time since death continues to be as big a challenge as it ever was. Duration of injuries is still a scientific guess. Forensic Psychiatry still subjective. Biochemistry of fluids has not become routine. This could provide immense objective data related to post mortem interval, injuries or cause of death in a few instances. Estimation of age of a person needs research to establish appropriate methods and to put in corrections in accordance with variable factors of an individual. Research needs to be done to assimilate data on drug addiction and estimate levels of drugs in a person in non invasive ways. Forensic genetics is yet to be researched.

A lot of sub specialties need to emerge and experts in each to make it realise its potential. Forensic Radiology has acquired the status of a separate branch in some countries and has helped in diagnosis of cause of death at these centres. It has established itself as the means to diagnose pathology in some cases, not possible in any other way. Forensic Dentistry, Forensic Anthropology, Forensic Histopathology all need to be developed and integrated with Forensic Pathology. Toxicology is very much part of Forensic Medicine but not functional in a practical way in most centres. The three main components of it Clinical Toxicology, Forensic Toxicology and Toxicology of Drugs of abuse need to be promoted. Poison information centre also needs to be established in a competent, accessible and accountable way.

Forensic Medicine people in the country needs to work on teaching skills too. Enhancing and upgrading teaching skills implies attracting good and motivated human resource to work in the field and make it reach higher levels of competence in a competitive spirit. It is about time to focus in attracting the right kind of people in larger numbers to this branch of medicine.

Integration with people in law in the modern age could simplify the working and save lot of useful time. Court evidence to distant places could be facilitated using conferencing system or perhaps Skype or similar methods. This could save lot of valuable time for the Forensic person, which could be used elsewhere more profitably. Travelling for court evidence to distant places may be entertaining but does take time and other resources as well. The quality of evidence needs to be directed to degrees of statistically substantiated opinion to prevent over opinionating or avoiding bias either random or conformational.

The infrastructure of Mortuary having better constructed and ventilated mortuaries and use of personal protective equipments for people working in the Mortuary could ensure safer working condition. Mortuary can be one of the most infected places and threat for infection could easily be high for mortuary personnel. The safety methods and good practices should be put in force in this area of the hospital too.

Working approach for autopsy needs to be protocolised so that quality of work can be standardised. In the era when intensive care units and surgeries are protocolised, autopsies should only be for all the advantages that would ensure.

The inhibition in sharing data ought to be minimised. Not all data is confidential. Autopsy data helpful for research should be made accessible to selected people for selected purpose on fulfilment of whatever data be assigned as required mandatorily.

The list of things required may look exhaustive when compiled and stated, but so it would be with any specialty where people may care to critically look and analyse.